Arnold's Way
RECIPE BOOK
ALL FAVORITE RAW FOOD RECIPES

Arnold's Way RECIPE BOOK
ALL FAVORITE RAW FOOD RECIPES

BY ARNOLD N. KAUFFMAN

EDITED BY BRIAN ROSSITER

ISBN: 978-1973976356

Photography by Brian Rossiter of Fruit-Powered.com and Megan Elizabeth of MeganElizabeth.com.
Book cover and interior design by Anna Chmielewska of AnnaCdesign.com.

First edition published in December 2014 by Arnold's Way.
Published in the United States of America.

NOTICE OF RIGHTS

MEDICAL DISCLAIMER

The information presented in this book does not constitute health, medical or any other kind of professional advice and is not intended to replace the advice of medical doctors or other healthcare professionals with whom you consult. You are responsible for your choices, actions and results.

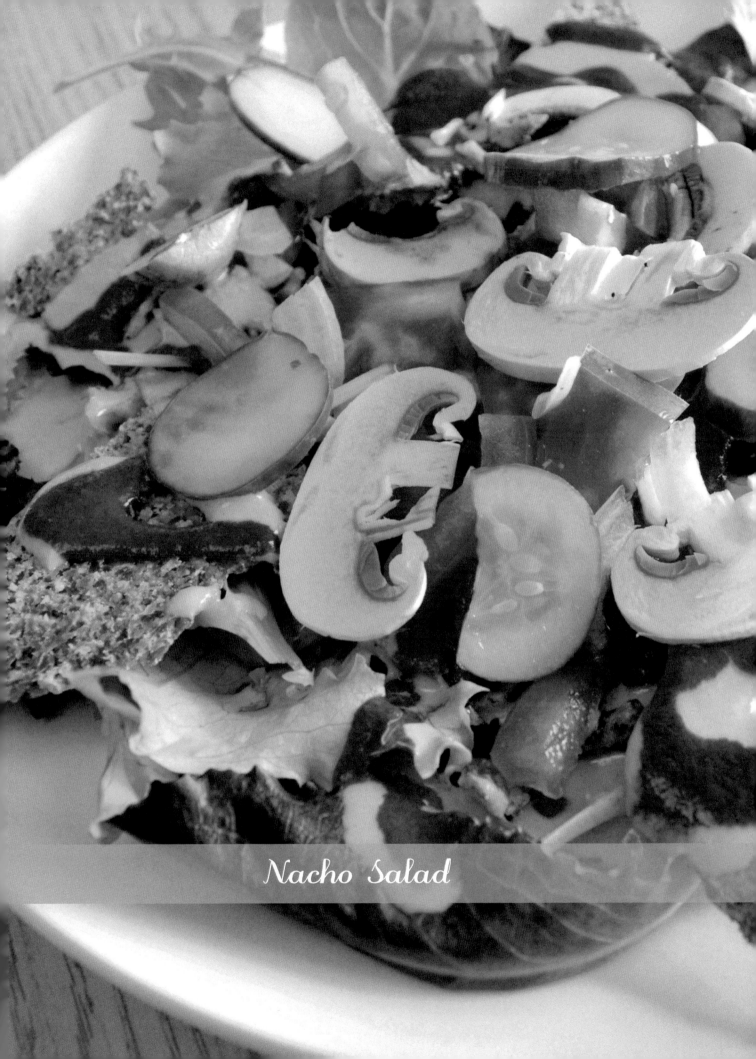

Nacho Salad

Foreword

I can't believe I wrote a recipe book. Well, I didn't. My daughter Maya did. In 22 years of business, I never really thought about making anyone food. In fact, knowing what I know, I would focus on selling fruit. It is on this note that the *Arnold's Way Recipe Book* came into being. Almost by accident and almost by choice. Almost as if a magical collaboration of high-powered indecisiveness came crashing together to make it happen.

Maya, who literally has been the main chef for most years at Arnold's Way, has been the deciding factor for most of the recipes and most of the day-to-day routine of creating delicious, mouthwatering entrées. In other words, she is the backbone of Arnold's Way, making it one of the premiere raw food cafés in the world.

Until 1998, Arnold's Way had been a vegetarian café for about four years. At the time, it was a go-to place for vegetarians and vegans, wannabe vegetarians and vegans, and those seeking a good place to eat at that was not expensive. I literally inherited the café. The previous owner had her second child and could no longer maintain it. While running a health food store after what had started as a vitamin shop, I reluctantly took over out of necessity more than choice.

What happened next would literally change the course of my life as well as Arnold's Way. In 1998, I took a self-improvement course in Natural Hygiene by Dr. T.C. Fry. Several chapters into the course, I was hit by an epiphany. I was hit in the head with a wild boomerang that had no place to go other than to me. I read that our natural diet should be fruit, and I was serving cooked food at the café.

T.C. Fry's words came across so strongly that I felt guilty serving cooked food. This was the beginning of Arnold's Way Vegetarian Raw Café and Health Center, as it is known today. I could no longer in good conscience serve cooked food. I had no choice in the matter. I let go of our chef and, with luck, prayer and Maya's work ethic, made it work year after year, struggle after struggle. Obstacles come and go. Arnold's Way has had its extreme challenges and superfun days. Our continuous goal is to create an energetic movement for the transformation to a disease-free world. It is our belief that, by changing your lifestyle one step at a time, this can happen.

We wrote this book as a way to help you create your dream as a raw vegan. Enjoy it and pass it on.

Keep the faith as I did.

Sincerely,

Arnold N. Kauffman

Summer 2014

Preface

I started working for my dad when I was 18 years old in 2002. No one taught me anything. My dad literally threw me in and said: "Here's the ingredients. Make the food." I started paging through books and tweaking dishes to create my own recipes, and that's how I learned about raw food. I'm all about fast, easy, simple and efficient recipes. If it takes more than five minutes to make something, it's too long.

One thing I love to share is how simple eating raw food can be. One recipe can be 20 recipes, only presented in different ways. My pies are literally interchangeable with one another. I tell my kids that the No. 1 ingredient in everything I make is love.

Throughout the 12 years I've been at the café, I have become more simplistic in my way of eating. Arnold's Way as a whole is becoming more simplistic. The healthier you eat, the more sensitive you get to simple recipes, and your taste buds explode with flavor!

It has been a wonderful experience working at Arnold's Way. Everyone who walks into the café brings out a part of myself I didn't know. When I meet someone at the store, I think, "How I can make the experience better for this person?"

I love being at the café, with everyone's beautiful energies embracing and helping me get where I am today. I have enjoyed truly beyond-incredible experiences with all my pregnancies and births. I credit this to working at the store and being surrounded by all the people in our community. I've raised my kids at Arnold's Way.

My favorite thing to do at the store is to peel bananas. It enables me to go into deep breathing, almost like a meditation. I learn to breathe in everything I do. I could breathe and just breathe. I'm heavily into deep breathing, visualization, putting my desires out into the universe, enjoying loving surroundings, eating and sleeping.

Family, of course, is my No. 1. I'm thankful for the support of my husband. I am beyond grateful to my dad, mom and family. I feel extremely blessed. I thank God every single day.

XO,

Maya

Arnold's daughter

Summer 2014

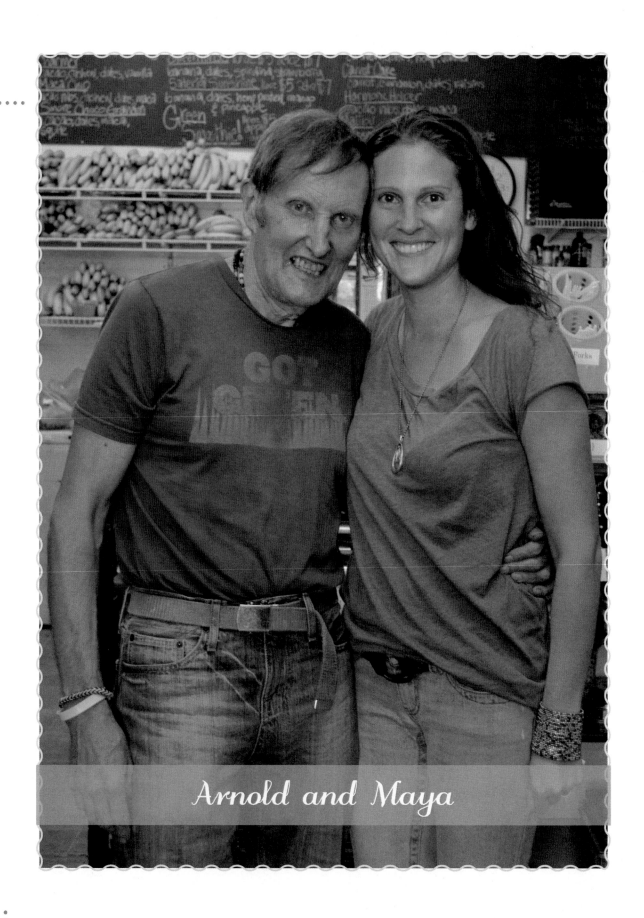

Arnold and Maya

"Every Moment
Is a Moment
of Love."

Notes from Arnold

I promote a mostly fruitarian diet that is low-fat raw vegan and involves no recipes. The recipes in this book may be used as a basis for changing your lifestyle toward a healthier you with the ultimate goal of achieving optimal health by maintaining a dietary regimen similar to mine. This book is a stepping stone in this direction.

On an average day, I eat, in the following order:

1. 5 BANANAS

2. GREEN SMOOTHIE (30 OUNCES)
   - 4 to 5 bananas
   - 1 pineapple
   - 3 ounces of dates
   - Greens (usually romaine lettuce)

3. GUACAMOLE
   - 2 avocados
   - 2 to 3 stalks of celery
   - 1 tomato
   - ½ cucumber
   - Juice of a lemon

4. BANANA WHIP
   - 5 bananas
   - 3 ounces of dates
   - 2 tablespoons of carob

I also graze on watermelon, blackberries, blueberries and other fruits in season until 6 p.m., when I generally stop eat eating. Three or four days a week, this is my routine.

For those seeking a pure diet, replace:

- Cacao with carob
- Granola with a mixture of dehydrated flaxseed, buckwheat, apple, pear and dates
- Maple syrup with blended dates and water
- Bragg Liquid Aminos or Nama Shoyu with coconut aminos or, optimally, lemon juice

And eliminate:

- Irritants such as salt, ginger, spices, garlic and onion
- Oil

Recipes made at Arnold's Way are often improvised using available ingredients. Recipe ingredient measurements are approximates.

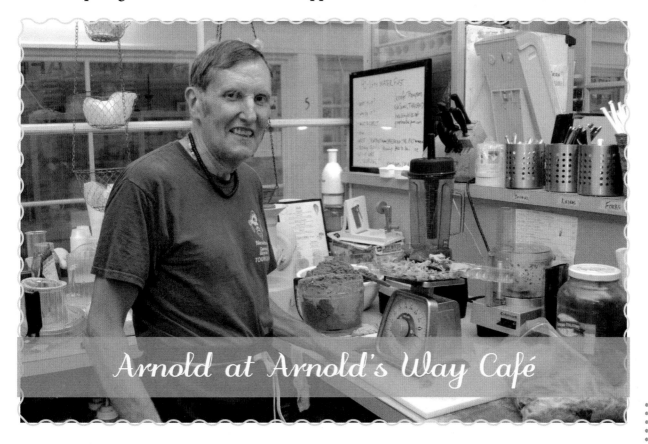

Arnold at Arnold's Way Café

CONTENTS

Smoothies

SERVING SIZE: 16 TO 20 OUNCES

...

Directions for All Smoothies

Break the bananas into thirds.

Core and/or chop other fruit.

For green smoothies, tear green leaves in half.

Add all ingredients to a blender and blend for 30 to 60 seconds.

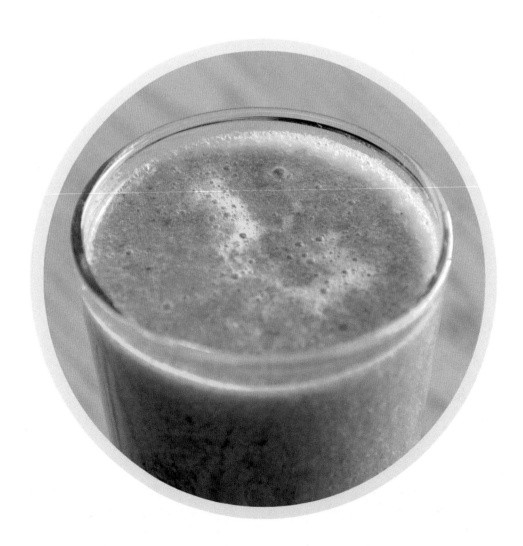

Green Smoothies

> *"Green smoothies are the basis for my daily dietary regimen," Arnold says. "They're nutrient- and calorie-rich and call for very little energy on digestion. In my opinion, they're the secret to good health."*

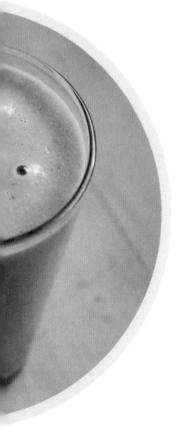

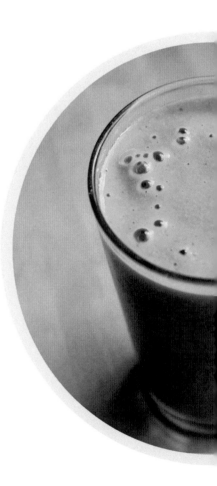

The Original Green Smoothie

2 bananas

2 dates, pitted

1 apple

1 pear

3 to 4 leaves of kale, collards or other greens

8 ounces of water

Green Force

2 bananas

2 dates

½ cup of strawberries

1 tablespoon of spirulina

8 ounces of water

Specialty Smoothies

...

Aloe-Berry

2 bananas

½ cup of strawberries

2 ounces of aloe

8 ounces of water

Berry Blast

2 bananas

½ cup of mixed berries (blackberries, blueberries, raspberries and strawberries)

1 tablespoon of goji berries

1 tablespoon of acai powder

8 ounces of water

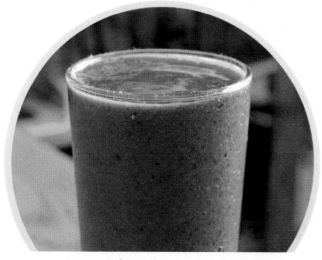

ARNOLD'S WAY RECIPE BOOK

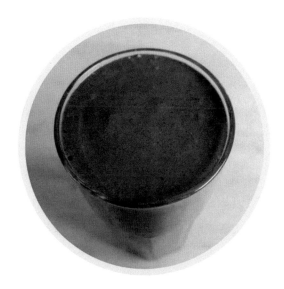

Carob-Berry

2 bananas

½ cup of mixed berries
(blackberries, blueberries,
raspberries and strawberries)

1 tablespoon of carob

8 ounces of water

Chocolate-Covered Strawberry

2 bananas

½ cup of strawberries

1 tablespoon of hemp seed

1 tablespoon of cacao

8 ounces of water

Simple Smoothie

2 bananas

½ cup of blueberries, strawberries,
mixed berries, mango, pineapple
or another fruit

8 ounces of water

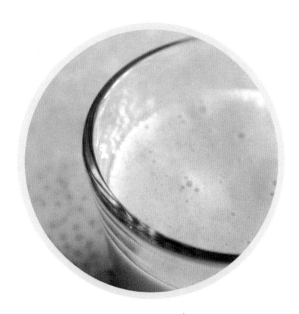

Piña Colada

2 bananas

¼ cup of mango

¼ cup of pineapple

1 tablespoon of dried coconut

8 ounces of water

Choco Charmer

2 bananas

1 handful of cashews

1 teaspoon of cacao

Dash of vanilla extract

8 ounces of water

Choco Maca Chip

2 bananas

1 handful of cashews

2 tablespoons of cacao nibs

1 tablespoon of maca

8 ounces of water

Warrior

2 bananas

1 tablespoon of hemp seed

½ tablespoon of mesquite

½ teaspoon of cinnamon

Dash of vanilla extract

8 ounces of water

Woodstock

2 bananas

1 tablespoon of carob

1 tablespoon of hemp seed

1 tablespoon of maca

Dash of vanilla extract

8 ounces of water

Sateria Sunshine

2 bananas

2 dates

¼ cup of mango

¼ cup of pineapple

1 tablespoon of hemp powder

8 ounces of water

Rainbow

2 bananas

¼ cup of mango

¼ cup of strawberries

1 tablespoon of acai powder

8 ounces of water

Juice Jams

SERVING SIZE: 8 OUNCES

"Have no more than 8 to 10 ounces per hour,"
Arnold says. "Otherwise, it's too much sugar for the body,
in my opinion."

...

Directions for All Juice Jams

If a recipe calls for ginger, lemons, apples or cucumbers, juice them before ingredients such as beets, carrots, celery or kale.

Carrot

6 carrots

Carrot Apple

4 carrots

1 apple

Blood Booster

4 carrots

3 celery stalks

1 garlic clove

½ beet

Daily Detox

6 celery stalks

2 kale leaves

1 cucumber

½ lemon

Rejuvenator

1 apple

3 carrots

5 celery stalks

Sliver of ginger

Green Machine

1 apple

1 cucumber

5 celery stalks

2 kale leaves

Sunrise

4 carrots

1 apple

½ beet

Sliver of ginger

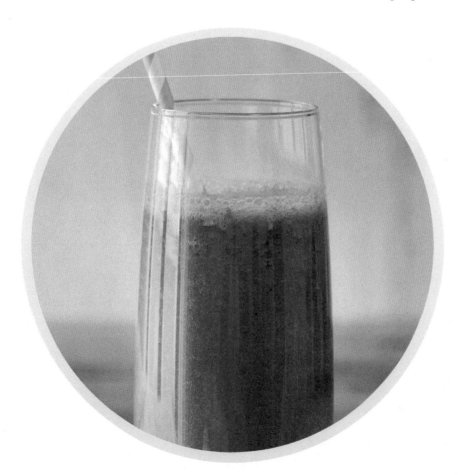

Banana Whips

A dreamlike concoction that's low in fat and one of the most popular recipes on the Arnold's Way menu. It's also Arnold's go-to dinner on almost a daily basis! A Champion juicer and its blank plate is recommended to make the best **Banana Whips**. You may also use a Vitamix blender or other high-powered blender or a food processor but are advised to defrost the bananas for 10 or more minutes before processing.

···

Directions for All Banana Whips

Use 4 to 5 frozen bananas, depending on size, per 16-ounce whip. Process the bananas and other fruits into a whipped form using a juicer and a blank plate, high-powered blender or food processor. Add additional ingredients such as fruits, nuts, seeds or powders to whips halfway through preparing them and top with the same additional ingredients.

"For a pure diet, use just fruit—no other ingredients," Arnold says.

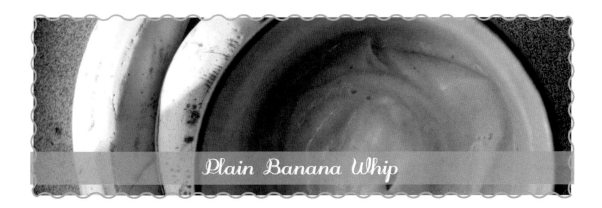

Plain Banana Whip

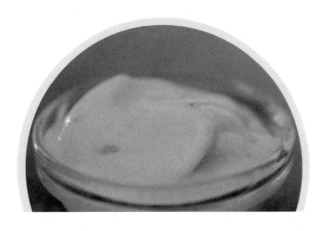

The Original Plain Banana Whip

4 TO 5 FROZEN BANANAS

Suggested toppings to design your own banana whip:

Blueberries, strawberries, mixed berries, mango, pineapple, dates, coconut, cashews, hemp seed, granola, cacao nibs, cacao, carob or maca.

Blend all ingredients and enjoy!

Extra

Date Caramel Sauce

8 ounces of dates, pitted
2 tablespoons of olive oil
1 teaspoon of cinnamon

½ teaspoon of sea salt
1 cup of water or as needed
to desired consistency

Tip: Sauce thickens when refrigerated.

Specialty Banana Whips

...

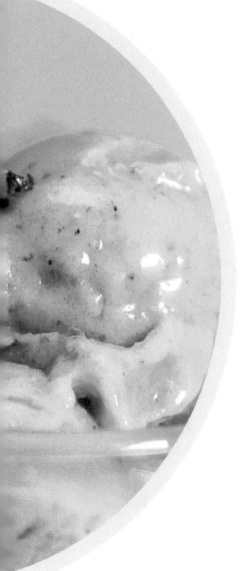

Banana Cream Pie

4 to 5 frozen bananas

3 dates

1 handful of cashews

1 tablespoon of hemp seed

2 dashes of vanilla extract

Carrot Cake

4 to 5 frozen bananas

2 tablespoons of raisins

¼ cup of carrots

2 dashes of cinnamon

Chocolate-Covered Strawberry

4 to 5 frozen bananas

½ cup of frozen strawberries

2 tablespoons of cacao nibs

2 tablespoons of cacao

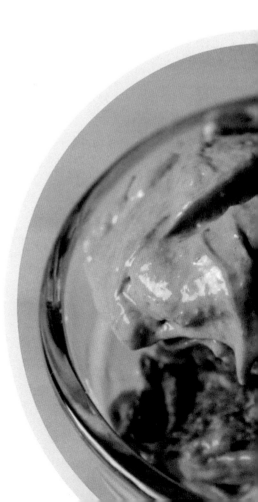

Chocolate Bliss

4 to 5 frozen bananas

2 tablespoons of dried coconut

2 tablespoons of cacao nibs

2 tablespoons of cacao

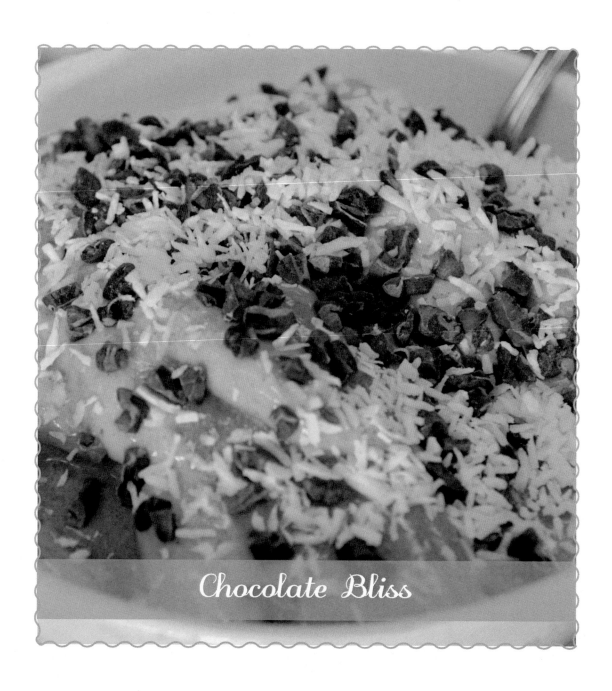

Chocolate Bliss

Caramel Crunch

4 to 5 frozen bananas

½ fresh banana

2 tablespoons of granola

Drizzle with *Date Caramel Sauce*

Malibu

4 to 5 frozen bananas

¼ cup of frozen mango

¼ cup of frozen pineapple

2 tablespoons of dried coconut

Fruity Tooty

4 to 5 frozen bananas

¼ cup of frozen mango

¼ cup of frozen pineapple

¼ cup of strawberries

Oatmeal Cookie

4 to 5 frozen bananas

2 tablespoons of raisins

2 tablespoons of granola

Dash of cinnamon

Hormone Helper

4 to 5 frozen bananas

3 dates

2 tablespoons of cacao nibs

2 tablespoons of maca

Superfood Crunch

4 to 5 frozen bananas

2 tablespoons of granola

1 tablespoon of maca

1 tablespoon of mesquite

Banana Whip Sundaes

...

Directions for All Banana Whip Sundaes

Peel and place one banana, sliced lengthwise, at the bottom of a bowl. Next, prepare a *Banana Whip* on top of the fresh banana using 4 to 5 frozen bananas. Process the bananas and other fruit into a whipped form using a juicer and blank plate, high-powered blender or food processor. Add additional ingredients such as fruits, nuts, seeds or powders to whips halfway through preparing them and top with the same additional ingredients.

	Bananas Foster	Chocolate Heaven	Strawberry Crunch
SAME BASE INGREDIENTS FOR ALL RECIPES	4 to 5 frozen bananas	4 to 5 frozen bananas	4 to 5 frozen bananas
	1 fresh banana	1 fresh banana	1 fresh banana
	2 tablespoons of dried coconut	2 tablespoons of dried coconut	2 tablespoons of dried coconut
	1 handful of walnuts	2 tablespoons of cacao nibs	2 tablespoons of cacao nibs
			1 handful of strawberries

Tip Drizzle with *Date Caramel Sauce*

House Recipe Ingredients

...

"House Dressing, Red and White Sauces, Toona and Cheddar Cheeze last 10 days refrigerated," Arnold says. "Bergers can last three to six months frozen, if not longer."

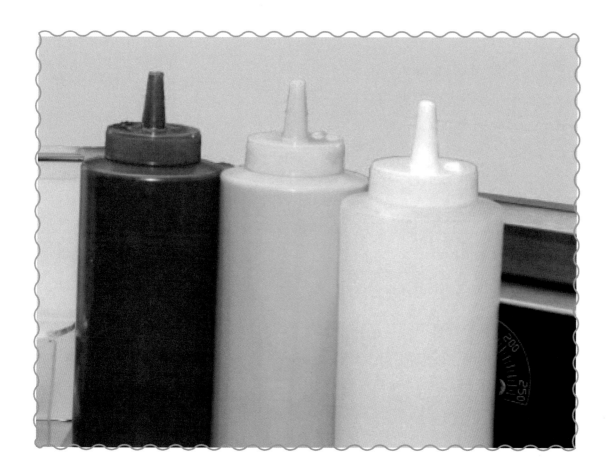

House Dressing

SERVING SIZE: 8 OUNCES

⅓ cup of Nama Shoyu soy sauce

⅓ cup of extra virgin olive oil

⅓ cup of agave

Combine all ingredients.
Cover and shake before use.

White Sauce

SERVING SIZE: 12 OUNCES

½ cup of cashews

¼ cup of sunflower seeds

¼ cup of Nama Shoyu

½ cup of water
or as needed to desired thickness

FOLLOW
THE SAME DIRECTIONS
FOR BOTH SAUCES:

Blend all ingredients to
a thin consistency and enjoy
on a variety of dishes!

Red Sauce

SERVING SIZE: 8 OUNCES

2 roma tomatoes

4 pieces of sun-dried tomatoes

⅛ beet

1 clove of garlic

1 ounce of olive oil

1 teaspoon of sea salt

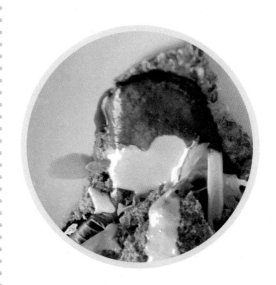

Raw Living Bread

SERVING SIZE: 8 SLICES

4 ounces of buckwheat,
soaked for 8 hours

4 ounces of flaxseed,
soaked for 8 hours

8 ounces of carrots, shredded

4 ounces of olive oil

1 to 2 tablespoons
of sea salt

Shred the carrots in a food processor. Mix all ingredients in the food processor, separating them into multiple batches if needed.

Apply the spread to dehydrator sheets and score four times to create eight pieces. Dehydrate at 105 degrees for 24 to 36 hours, depending on thickness.

Flip the bread and continue dehydrating for 12 hours longer.

When dried, break apart the pieces and enjoy alone, as bread for sandwiches and with salads or other meals!

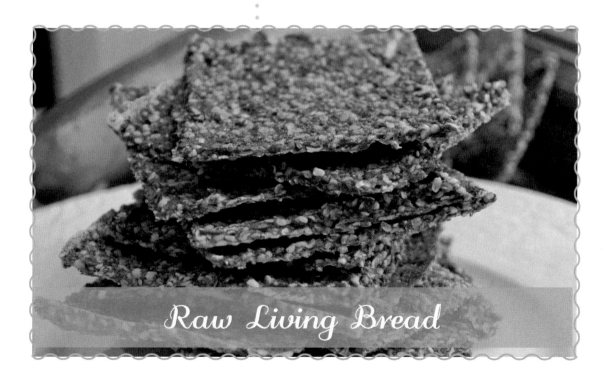

Raw Living Bread

Raw Berger

SERVING SIZE: MAKES 8 TO 10 5-OUNCE BERGERS

5 carrots, shredded

2 stalks of celery, chopped

¼ cup of flaxseed meal

½ onion, chopped

¼ cup of olive oil

2 tablespoons of cumin

1 tablespoon of sea salt

Mix all ingredients in a food processor, separating them into multiple batches. Apply mixture to dehydrator sheets and form patties about a half-inch in thickness.

Dehydrate at 105 degrees for 18 to 24 hours, depending on thickness, flip the Bergers and continue dehydrating for three hours longer.

When dried, enjoy with salads or other meals!

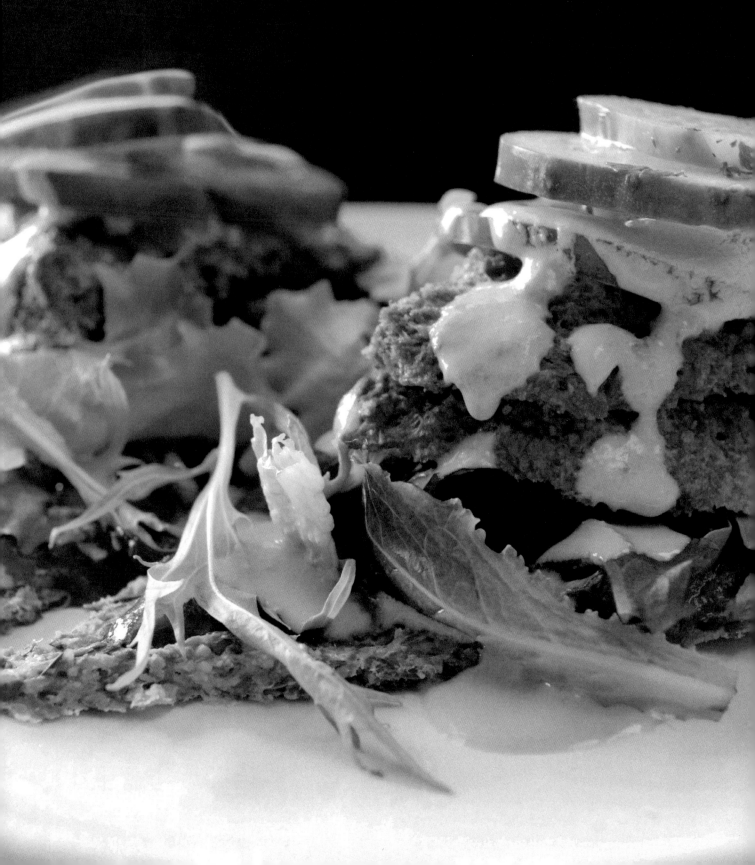

Cheezeberger Sandwich (see page 57)

Toona

SERVING SIZE: 12 OUNCES

Creamy base

1 cup of cashews

1 celery stalk

⅓ onion

1 teaspoon of dulse flakes

½ teaspoon of sea salt

Juice of ⅔ lemon

Chunky part

⅛ cup of carrots

⅛ celery stalk

2 pickles

Mix the cashews in a food processor. Add the rest of the ingredients for the first batch to the food processor and mix well, placing into a bowl.

Mix the ingredients for the second batch in the food processor until chunky. Finally, mix both batches in the bowl with a spoon and enjoy!

Try it with green onion, dill and oil! **Tip**

Cheddar Cheeze

SERVING SIZE: 10 OUNCES

1 cup of cashews

⅔ red pepper

Juice of ⅔ lemon

½ teaspoon of sea salt

Water as needed

Mix the cashews in a food processor. Add the rest of the ingredients and mix well and enjoy!

Appetizers

...

Small Side Salad

1 ounce of spring mix lettuce

1 broccoli floret, chopped

½ roma tomato, sliced

½ carrot, grated

½ avocado, chopped

2 ounces of *House Dressing*

Combine and mix all ingredients, enjoying over the spring mix lettuce!

Marinated Mushrooms

1 ounce of spring mix lettuce

10 button mushrooms, chopped

¼ red bell pepper, chopped

¼ yellow onion, chopped

1 garlic clove, minced

2 ounces of *House Dressing*

Combine and mix all ingredients, enjoying over the spring mix lettuce!

Half Avocado Sandwich

1 slice of *Raw Living Bread*

Lettuce to cover slice

½ roma tomato, sliced

½ avocado

Drizzle with *White Sauce*

Layer *Raw Living Bread* with lettuce and top with the avocado and tomato.
Drizzle with *White Sauce* and enjoy!

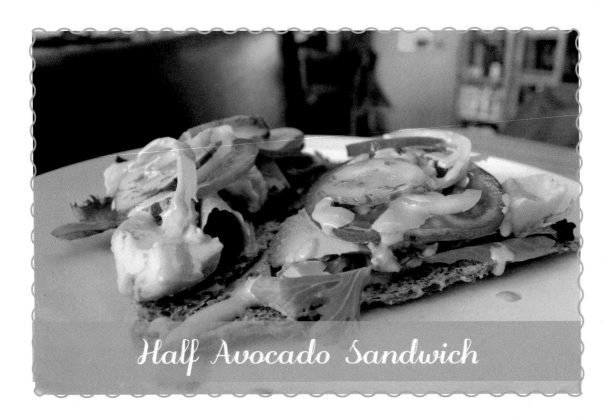

Half Avocado Sandwich

Raw Soups

...

Directions for All Raw Soups

Blend 7 to 8 ounces of fresh vegetables smooth with 7 to 8 ounces of water,
1 ounce of extra virgin olive oil and ½ ounce of coconut aminos!

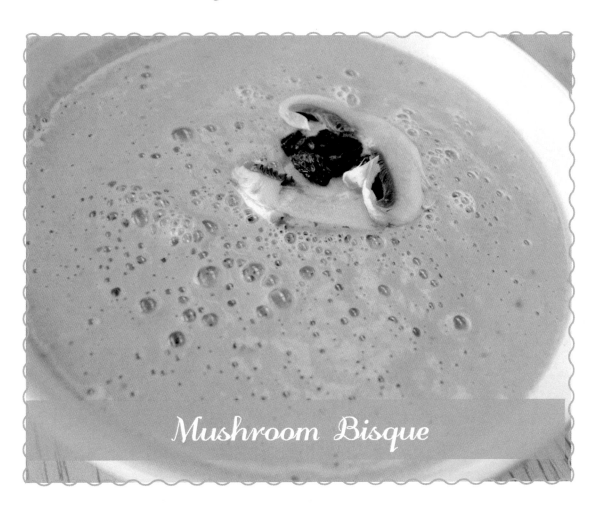

Mushroom Bisque

Mushroom Bisque

"This sounds off the wall, but it's yummy," Arnold says.

5 button mushrooms

1 ounce of cashews

1 ounce of raisins

2 garlic cloves

Borscht

"Just like mother used to make—only better!" Arnold says.

1 beet

3 carrots

3 celery stalks

1 ounce of sunflower seeds

Carrot Ginger Kream

2 carrots

3 dates

½ avocado

3 ginger slivers

Gazpacho

3 tomatoes

2 celery stalks

1 zucchini

½ red bell pepper

1 garlic clove

Tomato Veggie

3 tomatoes

2 carrots

2 celery stalks

½ red bell pepper

Rich Greens

1 zucchini

1 avocado

1 ounce of pumpkin seeds

½ cup of broccoli

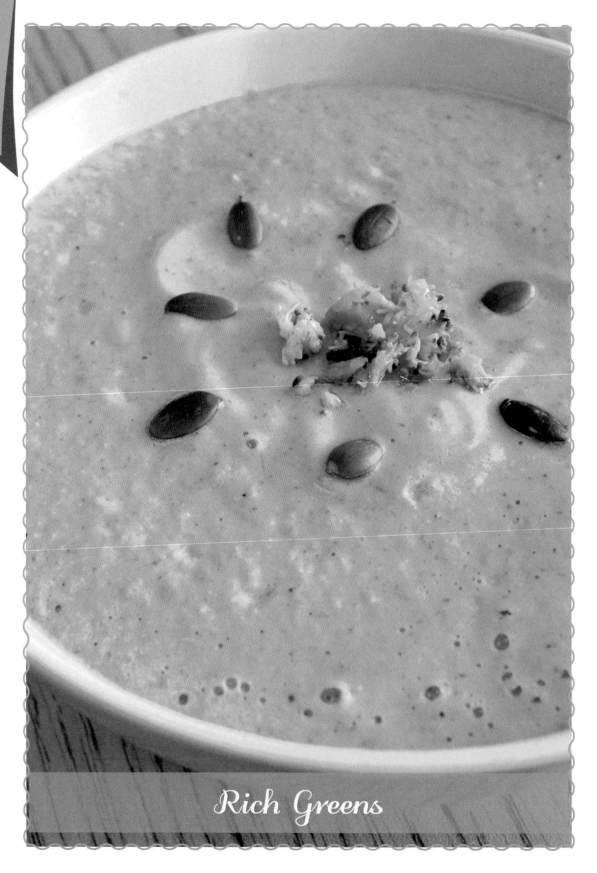

Rich Greens

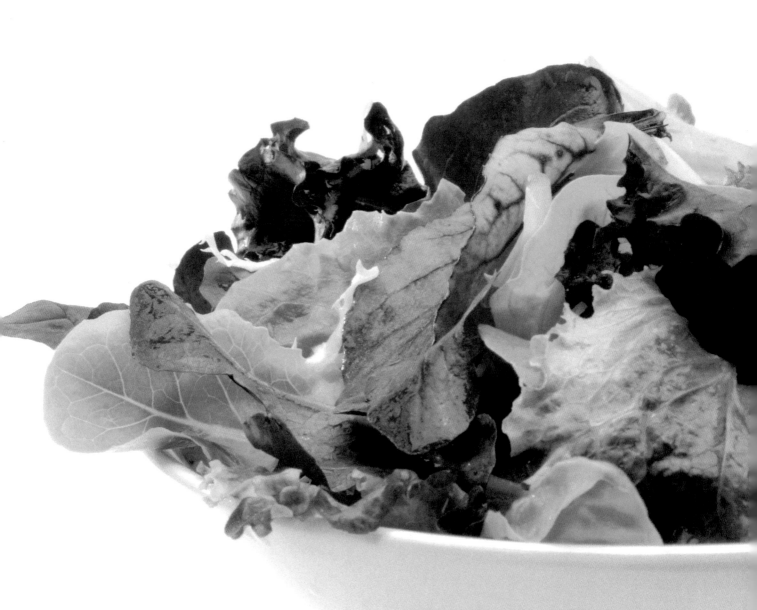

Salads

...

Directions for All Salads

Combine and mix all ingredients, enjoying over the spring mix lettuce!

Leafy Green Salads

*Organic greens with hand-sliced veggies,
served with House Dressing.*

...

Garden Salad

2 ounces of spring mix lettuce

1 broccoli floret, chopped

½ roma tomato, sliced

½ avocado

¼ carrot, grated

¼ cucumber, chopped

2 ounces of *House Dressing*

Avocado Salad

2 ounces of spring mix lettuce

½ avocado, chopped

¼ celery stalk, chopped

¼ carrot, grated

¼ yellow onion, chopped

1 tablespoon of pumpkin seeds

Apple Hemp Raisin Salad

2 ounces of spring mix lettuce

1 apple, chopped

2 tablespoons of raisins

1 tablespoon of hemp seed

Beet Salad

2 ounces of spring mix lettuce

½ apple, chopped

¼ beet, chopped

¼ carrot, grated

2 tablespoons of raisins

1 tablespoon of hemp seed

Berger Salad

2 ounces of spring mix lettuce

1 *Raw Berger*, crumpled

1 broccoli floret, chopped

½ roma tomato, sliced

1 button mushroom, chopped

¼ onion, chopped

Top with 2 pickles, chopped

Drizzle with *Red* and *White Sauces*

Nacho Salad

2 ounces of spring mix lettuce

½ roma tomato, sliced

½ avocado, chopped

1 button mushroom, chopped

¼ onion, chopped

Croutons from 1 slice of *Raw Living Bread*, crumpled

Top with 2 pickles, chopped

Drizzle with *Red* and *White Sauces*

Toona Salad

2 ounces of spring mix lettuce

3 ounces of *Toona*

½ roma tomato, sliced

¼ carrot, grated

¼ onion, chopped

Top with 2 pickles, chopped

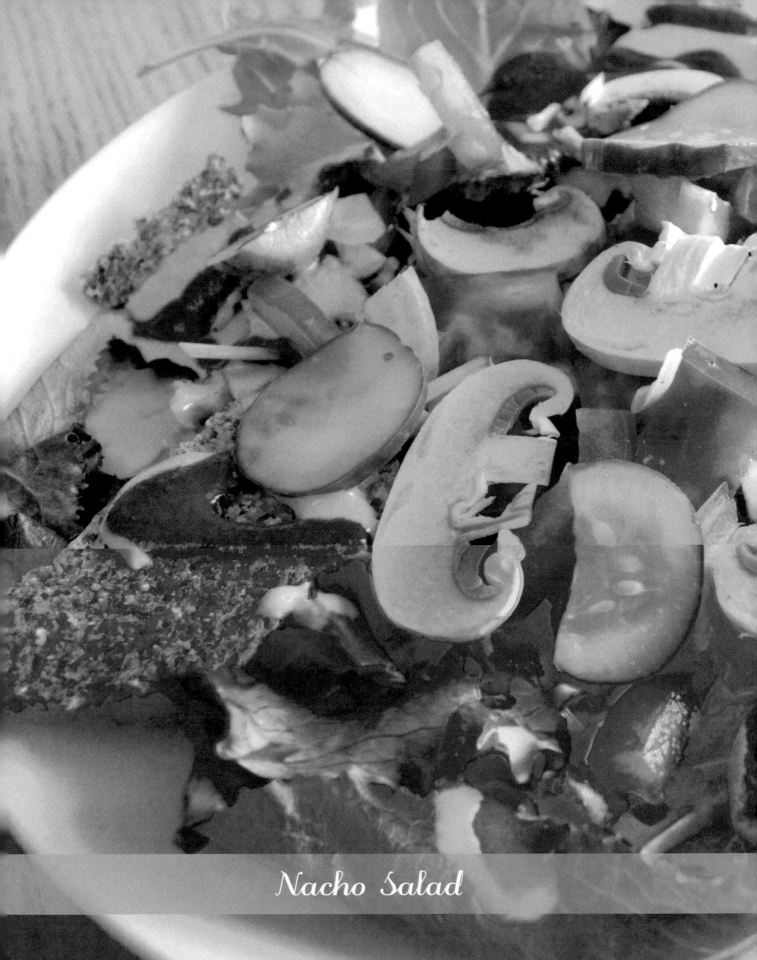

Nacho Salad

Chopped Salads

...

Directions for All Chopped Salads

Using a food processor, pulse chop all ingredients, comprising 8 to 10 ounces, other than greens and sauces and serve with a small bed of lettuce on the edges of the plate. Enjoy!

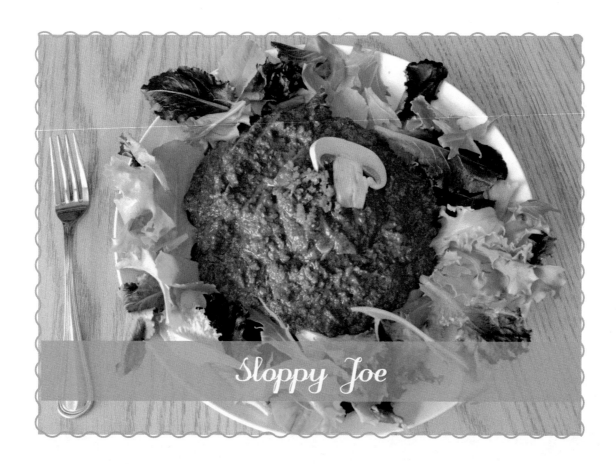

Sloppy Joe

Un-Chick

1 ounce of spring mix lettuce

½ celery stalk, chopped

½ zucchini, chopped

⅓ onion, chopped

¼ cup of mushrooms, chopped

4 olives

Drizzle with *White Sauce*

Sloppy Joe

"I love the Sloppy Joe," Arnold says. "I named it for Matt Goodman, who created it. It's very good, very tasty."

1 ounce of spring mix lettuce

1 *Raw Berger* patty

1 roma tomato, sliced

⅓ onion, chopped

1 garlic clove, minced

1 tablespoon of olive oil

¼ ounce of Bragg Liquid Aminos

Drizzle with *Red Sauce*

Kyle's Smile

1 ounce of spring mix lettuce

1 Raw Berger patty

1 roma tomato, sliced

½ avocado, chopped

⅓ onion, chopped

¼ zucchini, chopped

¼ cup of mushrooms, chopped

4 olives

2 ounces of *House Dressing*

Polynesian Delight

1 ounce of spring mix lettuce

1 roma tomato, sliced

2 Medjool dates, pitted and chopped

½ cup of mango, chopped

½ cup of pineapple, chopped

5 tablespoons of dried coconut

Zesty Salad

1 ounce of spring mix lettuce

1 apple, chopped

½ roma tomato, sliced

½ celery stalk, chopped

½ carrot, grated

½ avocado, chopped

Juice of ½ lemon

3 dashes of dulse

2 ounces of *House Dressing*

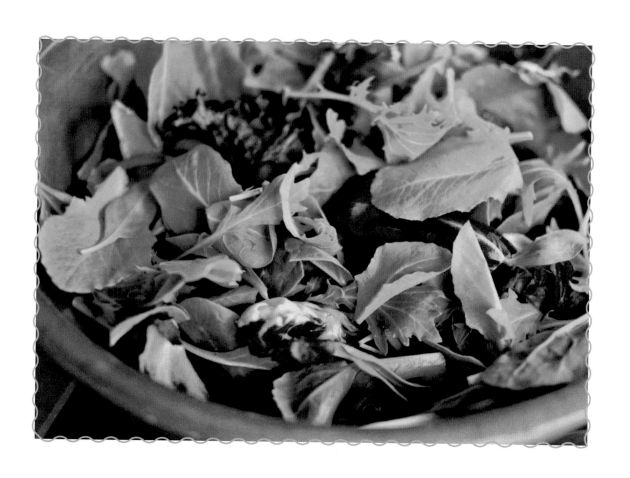

Entrées
Low-Fat Meals

...

Arnold's Special Low-Fat Spaghetti

"Low-Fat Spaghetti is my favorite go-to recipe for guests,"
Arnold says. "It looks good and is superdelish!"

1½ zucchini, ends chopped

2 roma tomatoes, sliced

¼ red bell pepper, chopped

¼ cup of mango, chopped

2 dates, pitted and chopped

1 Nori sheet

To make spaghetti, use a spiralizer to cut the zucchini into noodles.
Place into a colander to drain and then place onto a plate or into a bowl.
Using a food processor, pulse chop the other ingredients
and pour over the spaghetti.

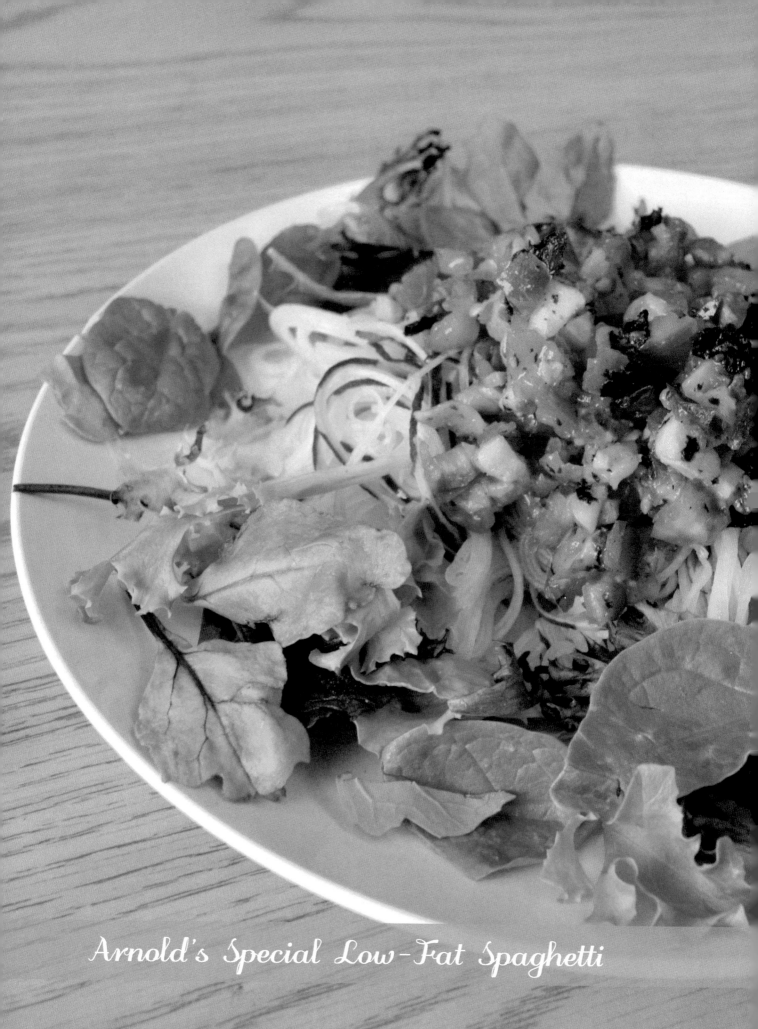

Arnold's Special Low-Fat Spaghetti

Apple Pear Delight

1 apple, chopped

1 pear, chopped

2 dates, pitted and chopped

¼ cup of raisins

3 dashes of dried coconut

Combine and mix all ingredients and enjoy!

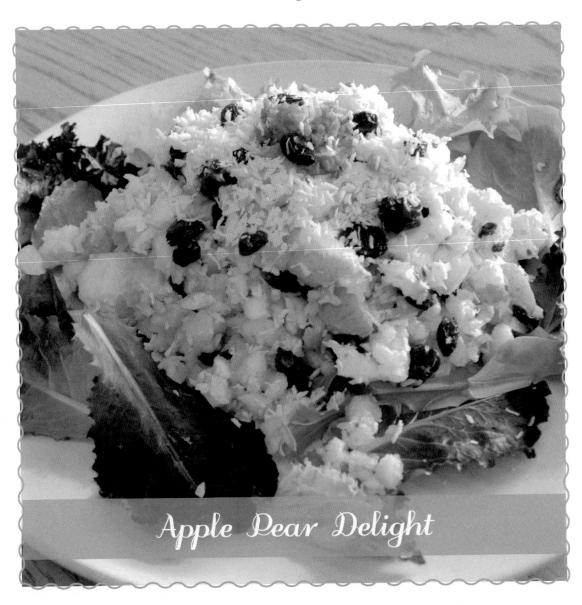

Apple Pear Delight

Banana Stacks

2 bananas

½ apple, chopped

½ cup of mixed berries

2 dates, pitted and chopped

Cut the bananas lengthwise and place onto a plate.
Using a food processor, pulse chop the apple, berries and dates
and pour over the bananas. Drizzle *Date Caramel Sauce* over the meal.

Banana Pancakes with Berry Sauce

4 dehydrated banana pancakes

½ cup of strawberries or mixed berries

2 dates, pitted and chopped

To make pancakes, dehydrate bananas liquified in a blender, food processor
or juicer. Blend the strawberries and dates and pour over the pancakes.

Carob Pudding

3 bananas

2 dates, pitted and chopped

2 tablespoons of carob

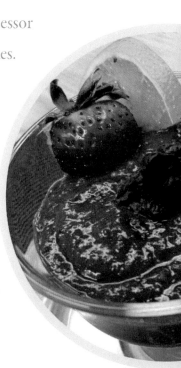

Blend 2½ bananas with the dates and carob and place into a bowl.
Add the remaining banana, cut crosswise into slices.

Arnold's Way Sandwiches

...

Directions for All Raw Sandwiches

Serve open face on two *Raw Living Bread* slices. Add *White Sauce* and then lettuce, followed by other ingredients. Drizzle with *White Sauce* and enjoy!

Avocado Sandwich

Spring mix lettuce to cover the bread

1 avocado

¼ roma tomato, sliced

¼ carrot, grated

¼ onion, chopped

Top with 2 pickles, chopped

Drizzle with *White Sauce*

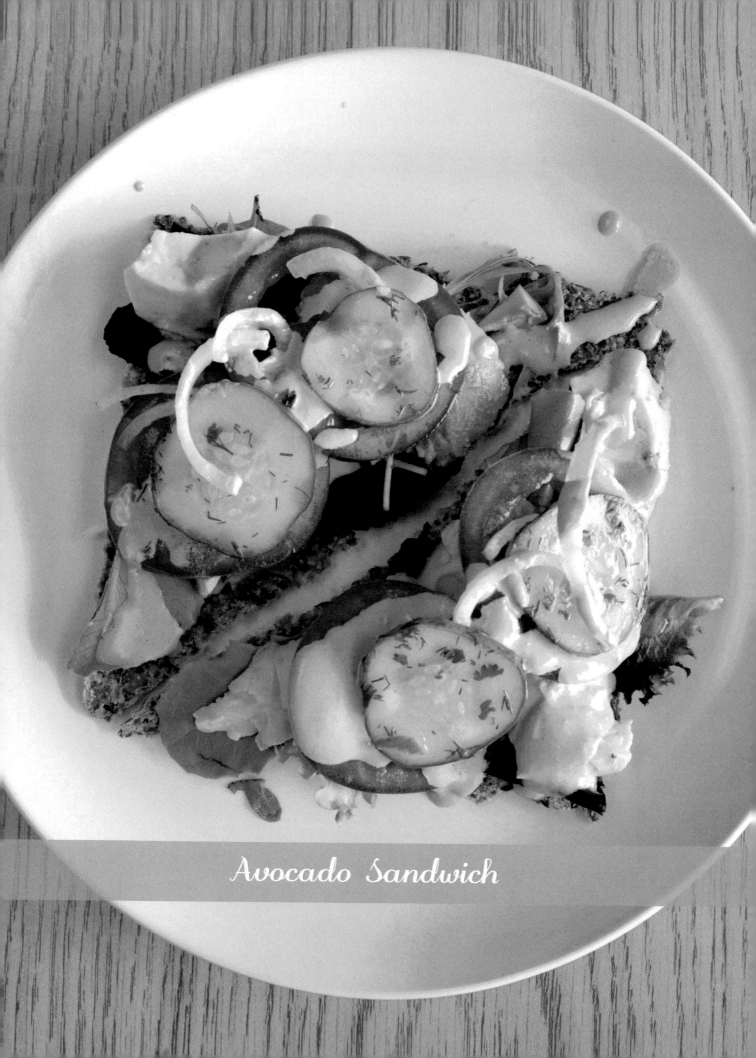

Avocado Sandwich

Cheeze Sandwich

Spring mix lettuce to cover the bread

3 ounces of *Cheddar Cheeze*

¼ roma tomato, sliced

¼ carrot, grated

¼ onion, chopped

Top with 2 pickles, chopped

Drizzle with *White Sauce*

Toona Sandwich

Spring mix lettuce to cover the bread

½ cup of *Toona*

¼ roma tomato, sliced

¼ carrot, grated

¼ onion, chopped

Top with 2 pickles, chopped

Drizzle with *White Sauce*

Cheezeberger Sandwich

(see large picture on page 33)

"This is my answer to McDonald's," Arnold says.
*"It's a no-meat alternative and what a real burger
should be made of."*

Spring mix lettuce to cover the bread

1 *Raw Berger* patty, cut in half

¼ roma tomato, sliced

¼ carrot, grated

¼ onion, chopped

Top with 2 pickles, chopped

Drizzle *Red Sauce* over the *Raw Living Bread*

Drizzle with *White Sauce*

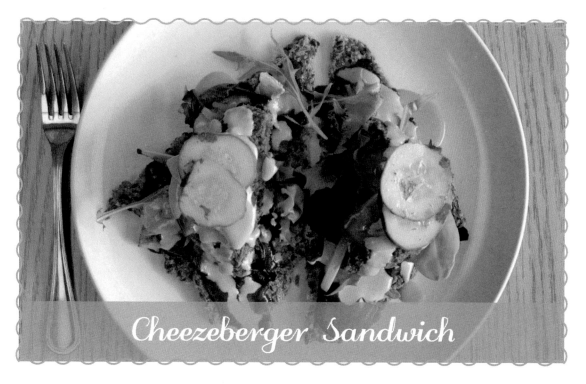

Cheezeberger Sandwich

Pizza & Spaghetti

...

Pizza

"This pizza is my answer to all those pizza joints with a crust that could make your mother proud," Arnold says.

2 *Raw Living Bread* krackers

1 roma tomato, chopped

1 broccoli floret, chopped

¼ cup of mushrooms, chopped

4 olives

Drizzle with *Red Sauce* over *Raw Living Bread*

Drizzle with *White Sauce*

Serve open face on two *Raw Living Bread* krackers.

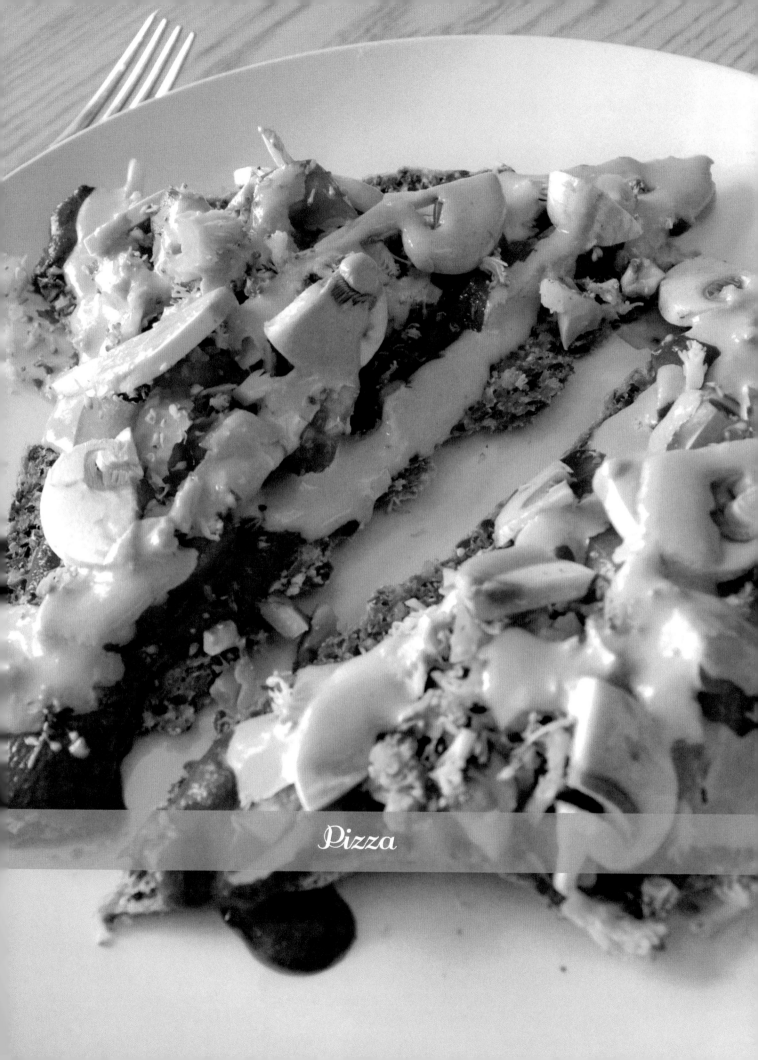

Pizza

...

Directions for Spaghetti Dishes

To make spaghetti, use a spiralizer to cut the zucchini into noodles.
Place into a colander to drain and then place onto a plate or into a bowl.
Process all remaining ingredients over the spaghetti and enjoy!

Spaghetti Alfredo

1 ½ zucchini, ends chopped

1 broccoli floret, chopped

1 clove of garlic, minced

2 dashes of oregano

¼ cup of *White Sauce*

Spaghetti Marinara

1 ½ zucchini, ends chopped

½ roma tomato, sliced

½ cup of mushrooms, chopped

1 broccoli floret, chopped

4 olives

¼ cup of *Red Sauce*

¼ cup of *White Sauce*

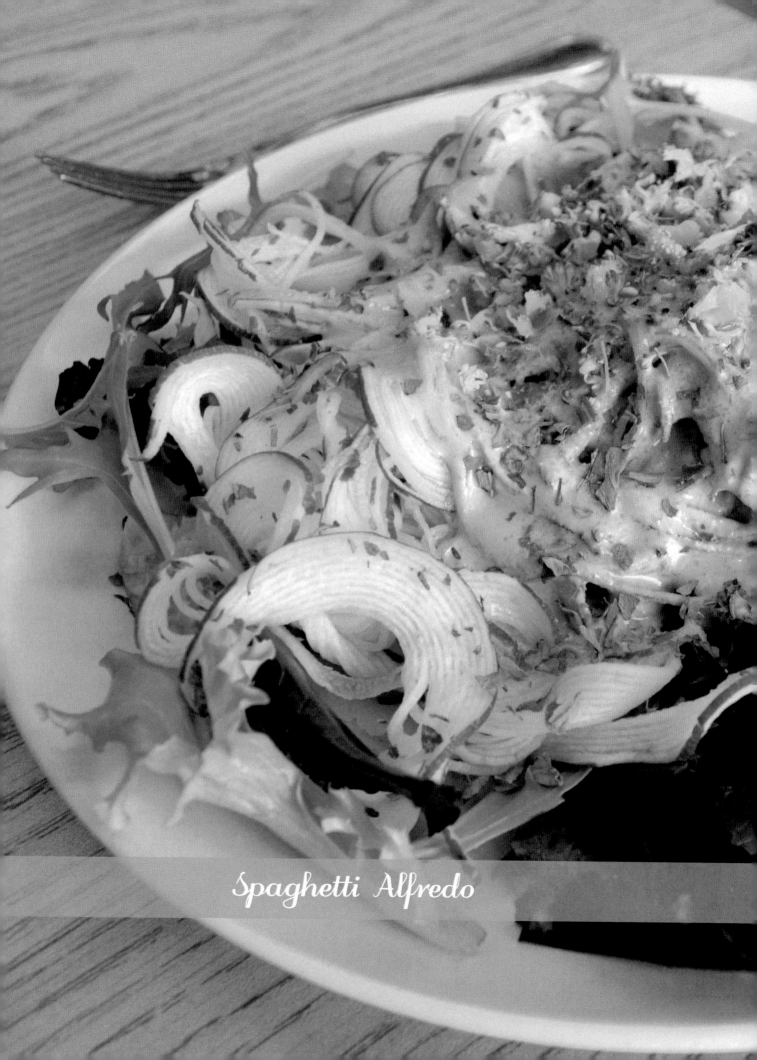

Spaghetti Alfredo

Nori Wraps

...

Directions for All Nori Wraps

Serve wraps rolled lengthwise with a small side salad. Add the lettuce first, followed by 8 to 10 ounces of other ingredients, pulse-chopped in a food processor. Enjoy!

Original Wrap

1 nori sheet

1 ounce of spring mix lettuce to cover the wrap and for a small side salad

1 avocado, chopped

½ roma tomato, sliced

¼ zucchini, chopped

¼ carrot, grated

¼ celery stalk, chopped

4 olives

1 ounce of *House Dressing*

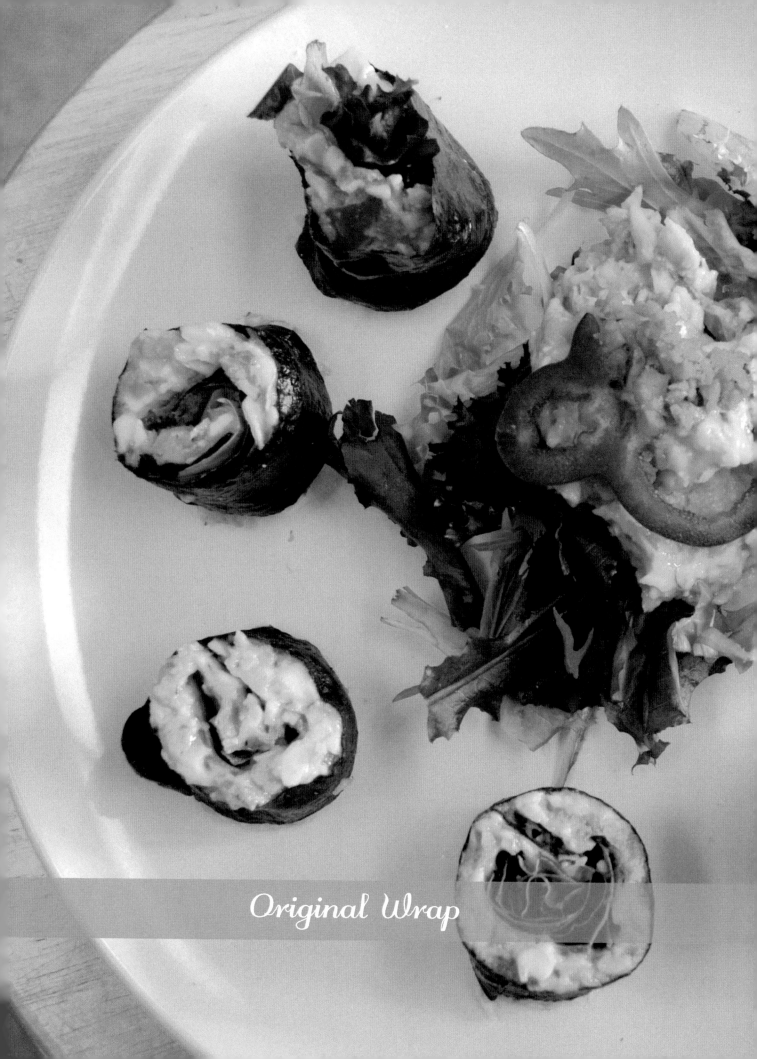

Original Wrap

Mediterranean Wrap

1 nori sheet

1 ounce of spring mix lettuce to cover the wrap and for a small side salad

¼ zucchini, chopped

¼ red bell pepper, chopped

¼ onion, chopped

4 button mushrooms, chopped

4 olives

1 ounce of *House Dressing*

California Nori Roll

1 nori sheet

1 ounce of spring mix lettuce to cover the wrap and for a small side salad

½ cup of *Cheddar Cheeze*

½ roma tomato, sliced

¼ carrot, grated

1 broccoli floret, chopped

1 ounce of *House Dressing*

Toona Nori Roll

1 nori sheet

1 ounce of spring mix lettuce to cover the wrap and for a small side salad

½ cup of *Toona*

¼ carrot, grated

¼ cucumber, sliced

1 ounce of *House Dressing*

Layer wrap with lettuce.

• • •

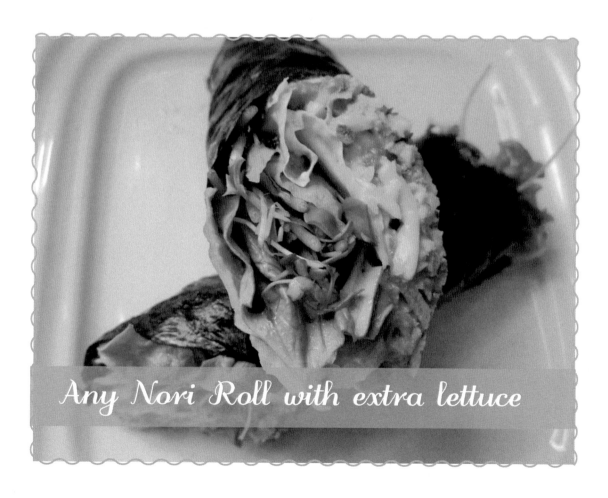

Any Nori Roll with extra lettuce

Bangin' Bundles

...

Directions for All Bangin' Bundles

Serve wraps folded into a square with a small side salad. Add the lettuce first, followed by the other ingredients, hand-chopped. Enjoy!

Avocado Bundle

1 nori sheet

1 ounce of spring mix lettuce to cover the wrap and for a small side salad

1 avocado, chopped

¼ roma tomato, sliced

¼ carrot, grated

¼ onion, chopped

2 pickles, chopped

Drizzle with *Red* and *White Sauces*

1 ounce of *House Dressing*

Berger Bundle

1 nori sheet

1 ounce of spring mix lettuce to cover the wrap and for a small side salad

1 *Raw Berger* patty, crumbled

¼ roma tomato, sliced

¼ carrot, grated

¼ onion, chopped

2 pickles, chopped

Drizzle with *Red* and *White Sauces*

1 ounce of *House Dressing*

Toona Bundle

1 nori sheet

1 ounce of spring mix lettuce to cover the wrap and for a small side salad

½ cup of *Toona*

¼ roma tomato, sliced

¼ carrot, grated

¼ onion, chopped

2 pickles, chopped

Drizzle with *White Sauce*

1 ounce of *House Dressing*

Cheddar Cheeze Bundle

1 nori sheet

1 ounce of spring mix lettuce to cover the wrap and for a small side salad

½ cup of *Cheddar Cheeze*

¼ roma tomato, sliced

¼ carrot, grated

¼ onion, chopped

2 pickles, chopped

Drizzle with *Red* and *White Sauces*

1 ounce of *House Dressing*

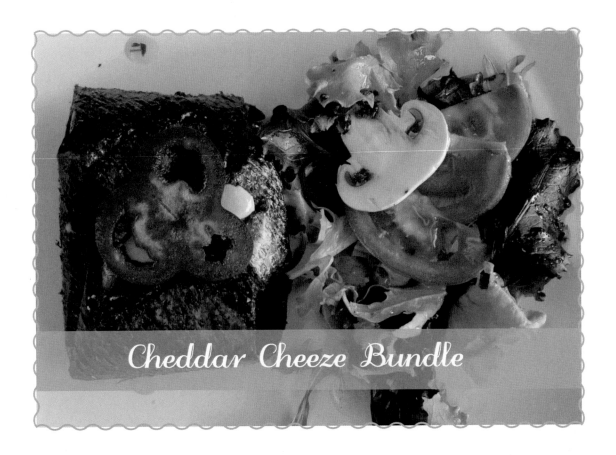

Cheddar Cheeze Bundle

Gorilla Wraps

...

Directions for All Gorilla Wraps

Serve wraps rolled lengthwise with a small side salad. Spread the *Cheddar Cheeze* or *Toona* first onto the wrap. Layer with lettuce and add the other hand-chopped ingredients. Enjoy!

Toona Wrap

1 large collard green leaf, destemmed

1 ounce of spring mix lettuce to cover the wrap and for a small side salad

½ cup of *Toona*

¼ roma tomato, sliced

¼ carrot, grated

¼ onion, chopped

2 pickles, chopped

Drizzle with *White Sauce*

1 ounce of *House Dressing*

Cheddar Cheeze Wrap

1 large collard green leaf, destemmed

1 ounce of spring mix lettuce to cover the wrap and for a small side salad

½ cup of *Cheddar Cheeze*

¼ roma tomato, sliced

¼ carrot, grated

¼ onion, chopped

2 pickles, chopped

Drizzle with *White Sauce*

1 ounce of *House Dressing*

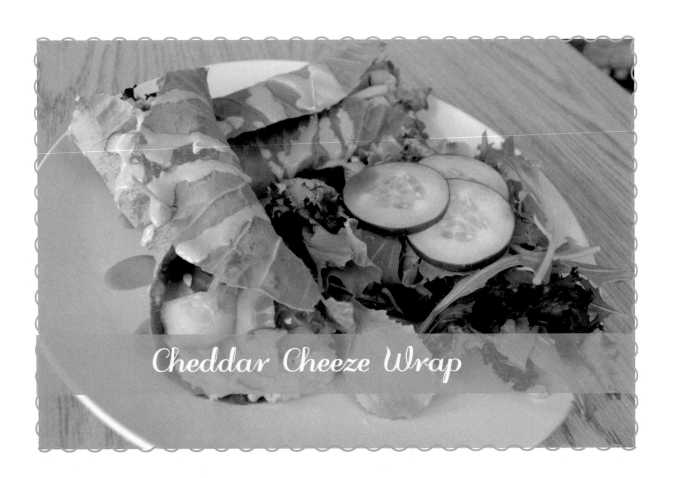

Cheddar Cheeze Wrap

Desserts
Amazing Raw Pies

...

Directions for All Raw Pies
unless specified otherwise

SERVE IN PIE MOLDS 6 INCHES WIDE AND 1½ INCHES DEEP.

Mix the crust ingredients well in a food processor.

Form the crust using the mixture in a pie mold.

Mix the filling ingredients in a food processor and place into a pie mold.

Blend the icing ingredients to desired consistency and pour over the filling.

Freeze and enjoy!

...

Carrot Cake

Crust

¾ cup of almonds

¼ cup of agave

½ teaspoon of cinnamon

Filling

1 cup of carrots, chopped

⅓ cup of dates, pitted

½ cup of cashews

⅛ cup of agave

⅛ cup of maple syrup

½ teaspoon of cinnamon

Icing

½ cup of freshly squeezed orange juice

¼ cup of cashews

⅛ cup of maple syrup

Start with *Directions for All Raw Pies* on page 71.
Sprinkle shredded carrots and cinnamon over the pie. Freeze and enjoy!

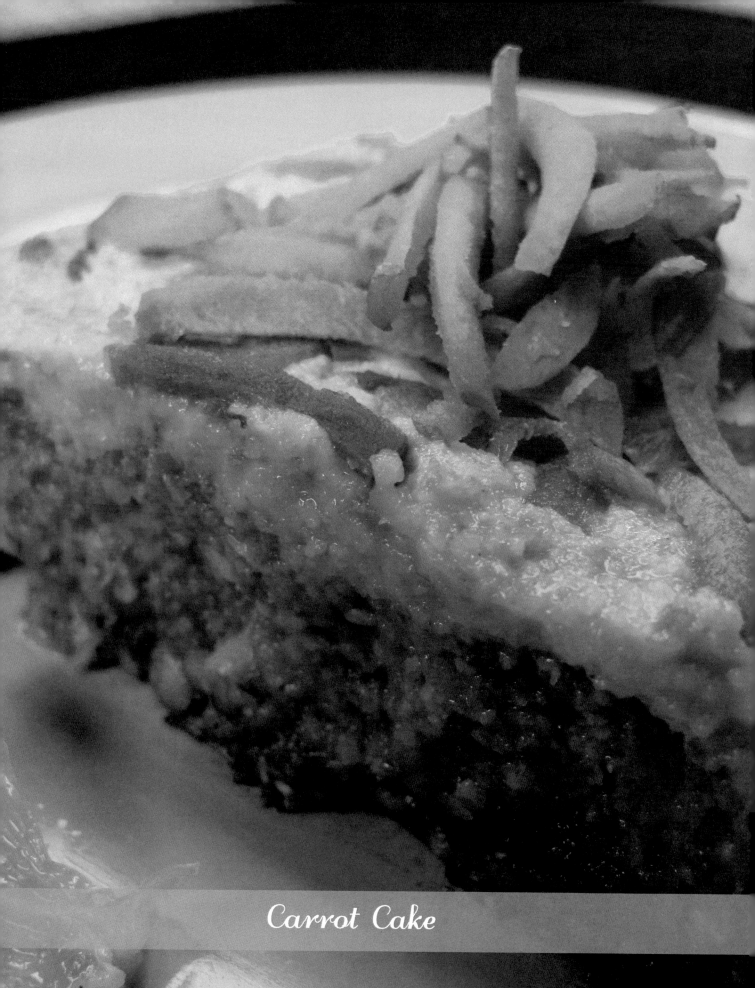

Carrot Cake

Chocolate Mousse

Crust

1 cup of coconut

1 cup of dates

Filling

1½ avocados

¼ cup of agave

¼ cup of maple syrup

⅛ cup of olive oil

⅛ cup of coconut oil

1 tablespoon of carob

1 teaspoon of cacao

½ teaspoon of sea salt

1 drop of vanilla extract

Follow *Directions for All Raw Pies* on page 71.

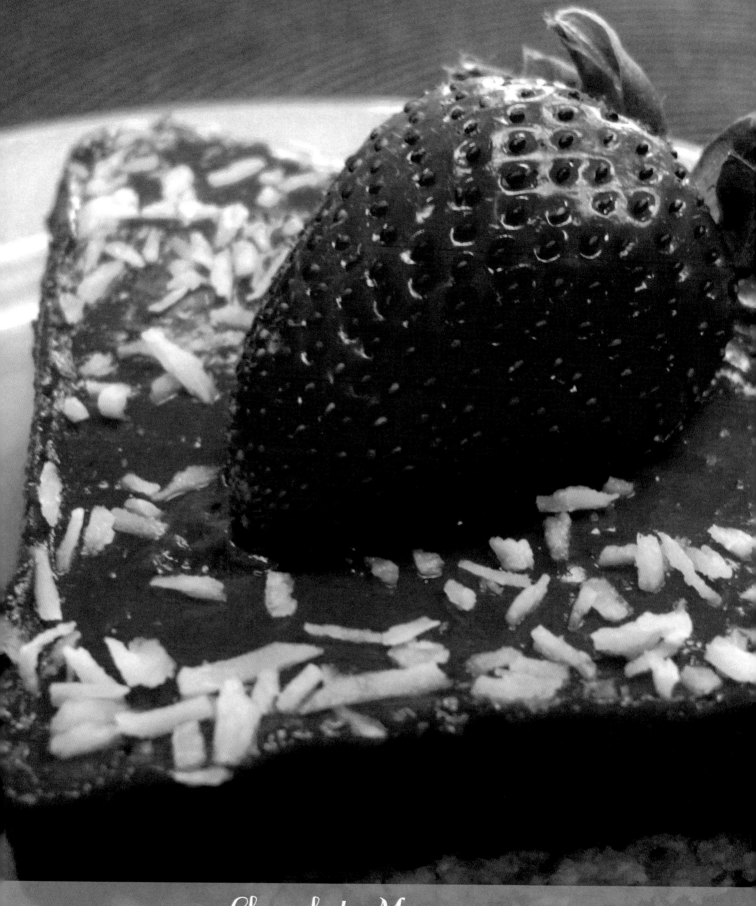

Chocolate Mousse

Apple Pie

Crust

¾ cup of almonds

¼ cup of agave

½ teaspoon of cinnamon

Filling

1½ apples, sliced thin

1¼ cup of maple syrup

⅛ cup of agave

⅓ cup of dates, pitted

⅓ teaspoon of cinnamon

Start with *Directions for All Raw Pies* on page 71.
Blend the filling ingredients and mix with apples. Pour over the crust.

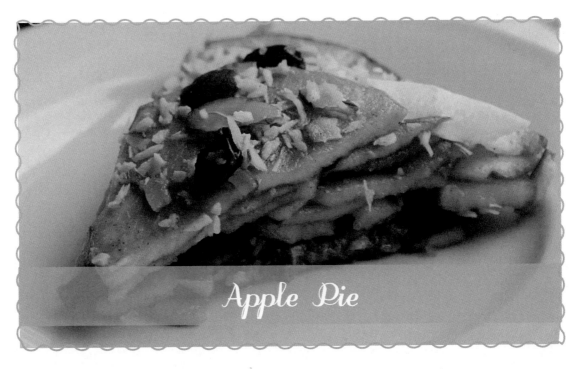

Apple Pie

Coconut Cream Pie

Crust

1 cup of coconut

1 cup of dates

Filling

1 cup of cashews

⅛ cup of olive oil

⅛ cup of coconut oil

⅛ cup of agave

⅛ cup of maple syrup

1 drop of vanilla extract

3 tablespoons of water

Icing

¼ cup of coconut, shredded

⅛ cup of agave

⅛ cup of water

Follow *Directions for All Raw Pies* on page 71.

Caramel Iced Cheezecake

Crust

1 cup of coconut

1 cup of dates

Filling

1 cup of cashews

⅛ cup of olive oil

⅛ cup of coconut oil

⅛ cup of agave

⅛ cup of maple syrup

1 drop of vanilla extract

3 tablespoons of water

Icing

½ cup of dates

1 teaspoon of cinnamon

1 teaspoon of vanilla extract

2 pinches of sea salt

¼ cup of water

Follow *Directions for All Raw Pies* on page 71.

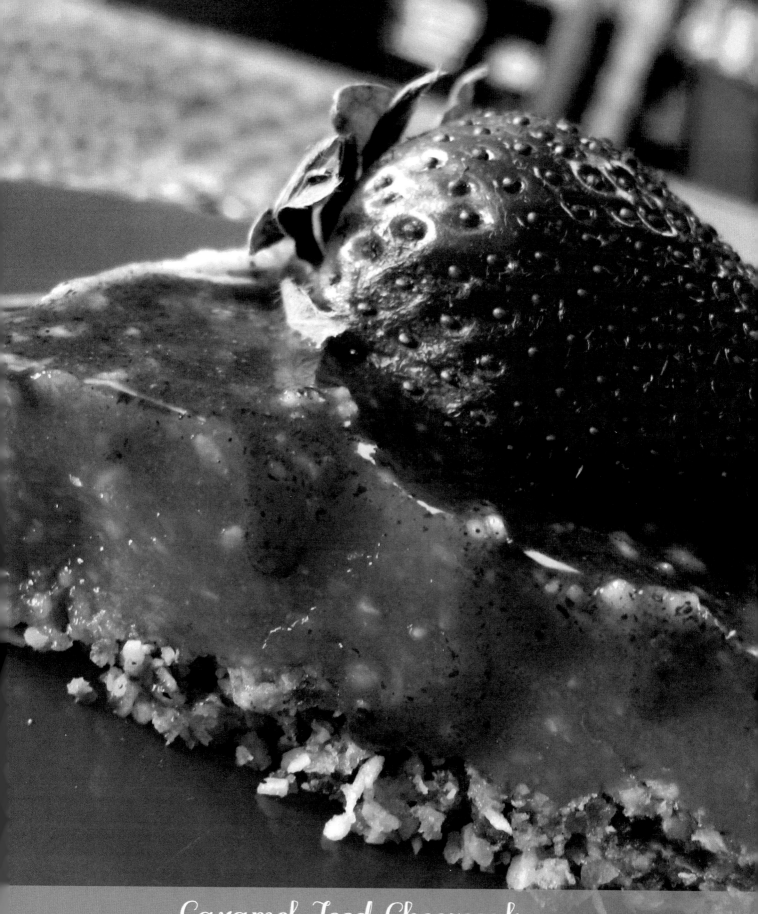

Caramel Iced Cheezecake

Blueberry Cheezecake

Crust

1 cup of coconut

1 cup of dates

Filling

1 cup of cashews

1/2 cup of blueberries

⅛ cup of olive oil

⅛ cup of coconut oil

⅛ cup of agave

⅛ cup of maple syrup

1 drop of vanilla extract

3 tablespoons of water

Icing

1 cup of blueberries

½ cup of dates

1 teaspoon of vanilla extract

2 pinches of sea salt

Follow *Directions for All Raw Pies* on page 71.

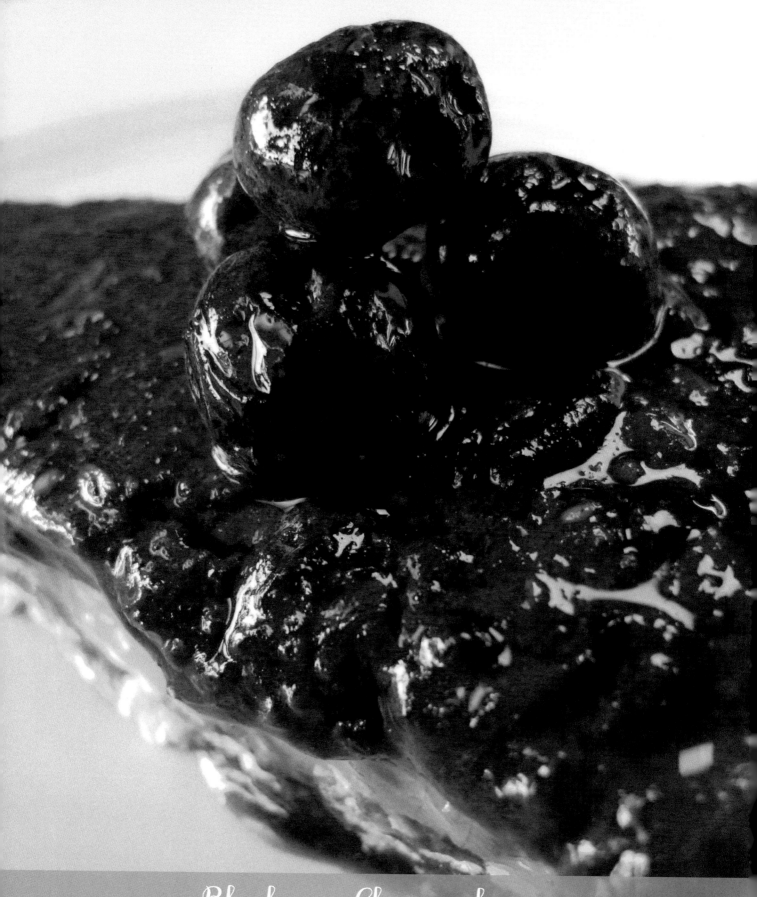

Blueberry Cheezecake

Carob Iced Maca Cheezecake

Crust

1 cup of coconut

1 cup of dates

Filling

1 cup of cashews

⅛ cup of olive oil

⅛ cup of coconut oil

⅛ cup of agave

⅛ cup of maple syrup

2 tablespoons of maca

1 drop of vanilla extract

3 tablespoons of water

Icing

½ cup of dates

½ cup of carob

Water to desired consistency

Follow *Directions for All Raw Pies* on page 71.

Potluck Recipes

"Potlucks are the key to building and keeping the community energy going," Arnold says. "What they do is bring everyone together for a night of education and to enjoy the food.

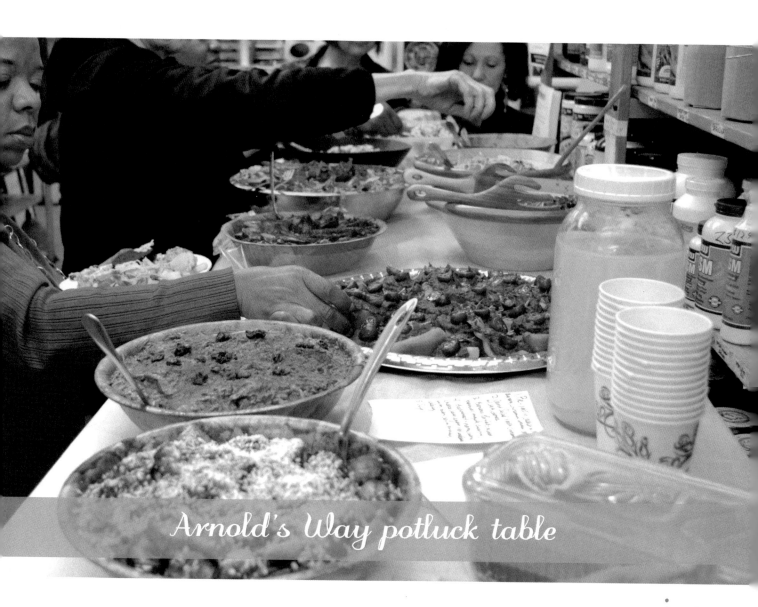

Arnold's Way potluck table

Salsa

5 roma tomatoes

½ cup of mango

1 red pepper, chopped

1 celery stalk

Pulse chop all ingredients in a food processor to desired chunkiness and enjoy!

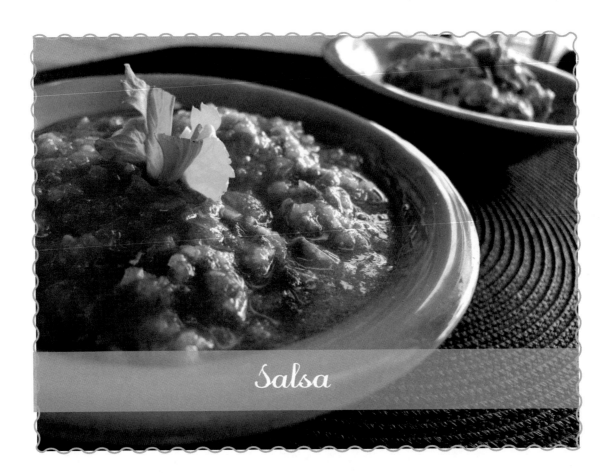

Salsa

Mashed Cauliflower

1 small head of cauliflower

1 cup of cashews

1 zucchini

2 cloves of garlic

2 teaspoons of olive oil

2 teaspoons of sea salt

2 teaspoons of nutritional yeast

Pulse chop the cauliflower in a food processor until smooth and place into a bowl.
Mix the rest of the ingredients until smooth and add to the bowl.
Combine well and enjoy!

Zucchini Orzo

4 zucchini

3 *Raw Bergers*

12 ounces of *Red Sauce*

1 ounce of cashews

1 ounce of nutritional yeast

Shred the zucchini in a food processor. Blend the rest of the ingredients
to create a hearty, gourmet tomato-Alfredo sauce.

Banana-Carob Pie Pudding

"This is my specialty for our potlucks," Arnold says.
"It's especially for the fruit eaters."

9 bananas

3 dates

6 teaspoons of carob

Dashes of dried coconut

Blend 2 bananas with 1 date and 2 teaspoons of carob and spread
in a midsize tray. Slice 1 banana crosswise and top spread.
Repeat this process two more times and top with dried coconut.

Raisin Pudding

3 cups of raisins

2 bananas

1 avocado

1 cup of carob

½ cup dates

½ cup of maple syrup

½ cup of agave

¼ cup of olive oil

1 tablespoon of salt

1 teaspoon of vanilla extract

Pulse chop all ingredients in a food processor until smooth.

Separate ingredients from the first and second batches into multiple batches, if needed.

Tip

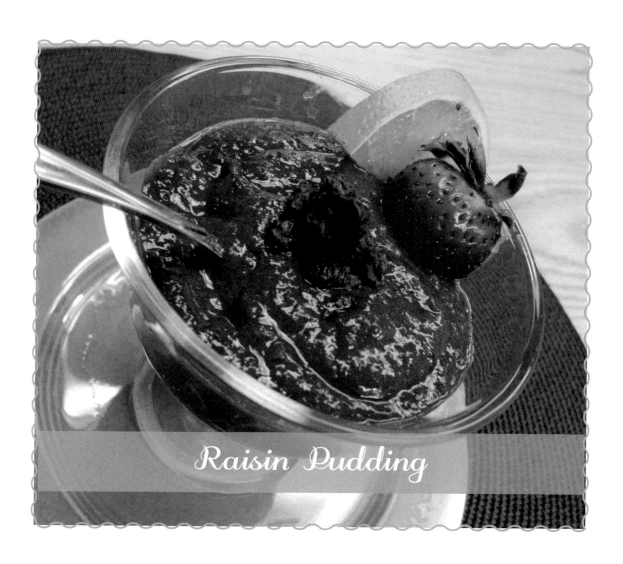

Raisin Pudding

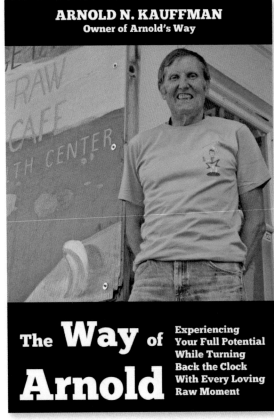

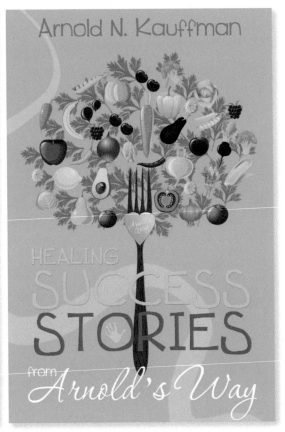

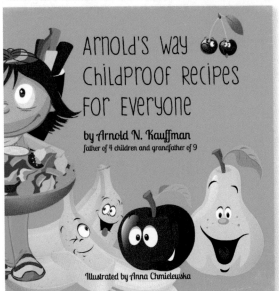

All books and films are available for purchase at Arnold's Way and online: Fruit-Powered.com/store.

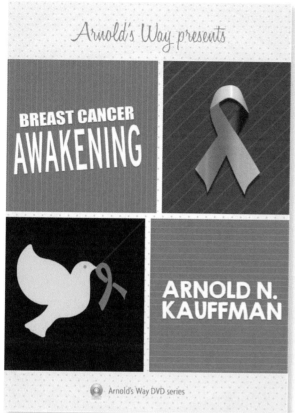

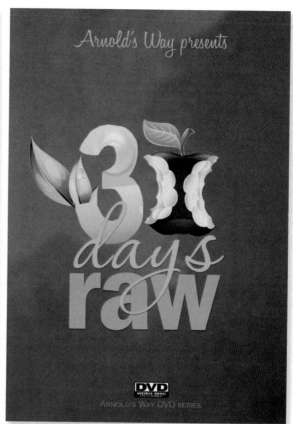

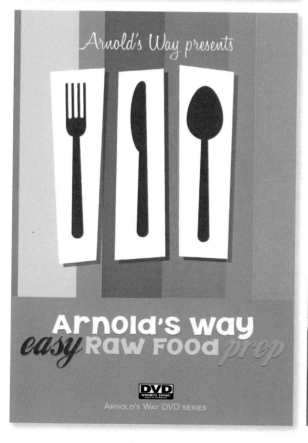

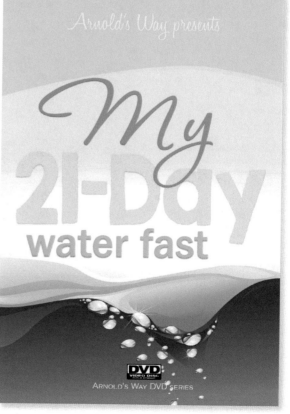

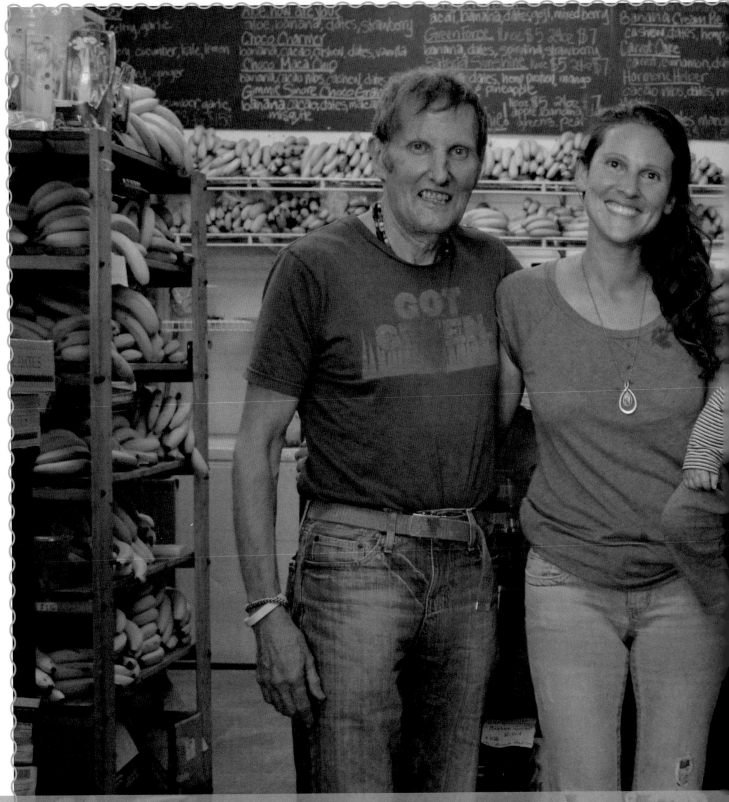

Arnold with Maya

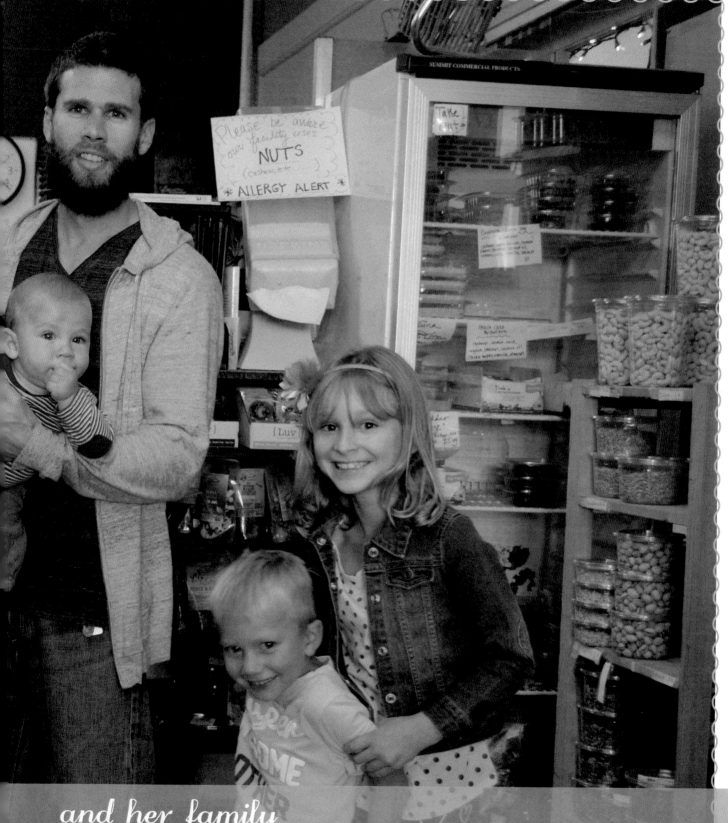

and her family

41093629R00053